My Doctor Appointment Log Book & Journal

THE PATIENT'S TOOL TO PREPARE FOR AND RECORD WHAT HAPPENS AT EVERY DOCTOR VISIT

Olivia Davenport

Disclaimer

Dedication

To patients everywhere, who are doing their best to work with their doctors to manage their medical care.

My Doctor Appointment Log Book & Journal:
THE PATIENT'S TOOL TO PREPARE FOR AND RECORD
WHAT HAPPENS AT EVERY DOCTOR VISIT

This Book Belongs To:

_____

If Found, Please Call or E-mail:

_____ or _____

Contents

Introduction

When I was a young adult in the 1980s, going to the doctor was a calm and nurturing experience. I never felt rushed or unimportant. I never felt like I had to remind the doctor of who I was or why I was there. Back then, I relied on the doctor to lead the way when it came to managing my health.

Fast forward to today. Going to the doctor is a very different experience for many of us. Not only do we often have to wait upwards of a month or more to get an appointment, we also have to deal with whirlwind visits because many doctors are only allotted 10 to 15 minutes for each patient. By the time it's all said and done, our appointment is over, and we leave the doctor's office with more questions than answers.

As someone living with a chronic autoimmune disease as well as recovering from breast cancer, I go to the doctor's office several times a month. I have found that my doctor visits are less stressful and more productive when I am organized and prepared.

For several years now, I have been using a doctor visit form that I developed for myself. Prior to each appointment, I would sit down and write out all my questions and thoughts to discuss with the doctor on this form. Then, I would take the form with me to the appointment, where I would ask the doctor my questions and write down their responses, plans for my treatment, and instructions for follow-up care.

That form helped me get organized and prepared for the few precious minutes I had with my doctor. At the same time, it helped with my anxiety about going to the doctor and feeling rushed while I was there.

In turn, and unexpectedly, it helped my doctors feel at ease with how to deal with me as a patient. My neurologist even asked me for a copy to share with his patients. And that's how the idea for this book came about. If this form has helped me over the years, surely it will be helpful to other patients.

Thus, *My Doctor Appointment Log Book and Journal: The Patient's Tool to Prepare for and Record What Happens at Every Doctor Visit* was born. This book is not just pages of blank forms, it contains helpful information about how to prepare for your doctor's appointment, tips for a productive doctor-patient relationship, an all-inclusive, fillable medical summary, as well as comprehensive and easy-to-follow doctor visit journal pages to be filled out prior to, during, and after each appointment with your doctor.

With this book, I hope you become empowered to work with your doctors to manage your medical needs and goals.

All the Best,

Olivia

Olivia Davenport

How to Use This Book

The purpose of this book is to help you prepare for and keep track of what happens during your doctor appointments so that you can get the benefit of managing your own healthcare.

Part I: Get Ready for Your Doctor Appointment

This section provides you with:

- Tips and checklists for getting organized and preparing for your appointment.

- Tips for how to maintain a productive relationship with your doctor.

Part II: Summarize Your Medical History

This section includes a set of *My Medical Summary* pages for you to keep up to date and ready for each visit. On these pages, fill in:

- Your contact information, including an emergency contact.

- Your medical history, including your medical diagnoses; chronic conditions and symptoms; any current medications you're taking; allergies to medications, foods, etc.; and past surgeries, hospitalizations, and emergency room (ER) visits.

Included at the end of this section is a *List of My Doctors* for you to add your doctors' names and specialities, as well as their addresses and telephone numbers for easy reference.

Part III: Record Your Doctor Visit Details

This section is where you 1) get detailed about what you want to accomplish during your upcoming doctor appointment; and 2) record what happens:

- *Table of Doctor Appointment Dates.* This is where you enter the date of the doctor appointment that corresponds with the *Doctor Visit Detail & Journal* page you'll be filling out for your appointment. This will help you easily refer back to the corresponding page of this book if you need to review notes from a previous appointment.

- *Doctor Visit Details & Journal Pages.* There are four journal pages for each appointment or visit with your doctor.

The following sections are to be filled out BEFORE your appointment:

- *Name of Doctor / Practitioner:* Write in the doctor's name or the name of the nurse practitioner, physician's assistant, or other medical professional you're seeing at the appointment.

- *Medical Specialty:* Write the specialty of the doctor, such as internist, family doctor, general surgeon, oncologist, rheumatologist, etc.

- *Appointment Date and Time:* Write the date and time of your appointment.

- *Reason for Visit:* Select either follow-up, initial consult, or other. If other, write the reason for the appointment.

- *Today's Symptoms / Concerns:* List your symptoms and any issues you are concerned about here.

- *Questions / Topics to Discuss:* Write your questions and/or topics that you want to discuss with your doctor. For each visit, there is enough room for five questions or topics. List them in order of importance to you. If you have more than five questions, you can write them in the *My Reminders / Thoughts / Notes* section of the form. Just be aware of and sympathetic to the doctor's time and ask if it's okay to continue beyond just a few questions.

The following sections (with gray background) are to be filled out DURING and immediately AFTER your appointment:

- *Vital Signs:* Enter your vital signs measured during the appointment, such as blood pressure, pulse/heart rate, temperature, and weight.

- *Answer To #:* For each of your questions/topics (#1, #2, #3, etc.), write in doctor's / practitioner's corresponding answers in these sections.

- *Doctor's / Practitioner's Instructions, Diagnosis & Action Plan for Me:* In this section, write your doctor's/practitioner's instructions for follow-up care, as well as the name(s) of any new medication(s) that he or she prescribes during the appointment. Also, write the date and time of any scheduled follow-up appointments.

- *My Reminders / Thoughts / Notes:* Here's where you keep your journal and write about important points your doctor makes, as well as thoughts and reminders for yourself about what happened at the appointment.

Part I

Get Ready for Your Doctor Appointment

The best patient is an involved patient.

ANONYMOUS

How to Prepare for Your Doctor Appointment

To have a successful visit with your doctor, you have to take a few minutes to prepare for your appointment. This means gathering information and taking certain steps so that you are able to quickly and efficiently share the most current and pertinent information with your doctor. This will enable him or her to give you the best care based on facts you provide, not speculation.

With this in mind, here are my checklists of what to do: 1) in the days and weeks before your appointment; 2) on the day of your appointment; 3) during your visit; and 4) after your appointment:

In the Days and Weeks Before the Appointment

- Ask the doctor's office for all required office forms ahead of the appointment so that you can fill them out at home, prior to going into the doctor's office. You may have the option of downloading the forms from their website, or they may mail them to you.

- Discuss the health insurance and payment policies of the doctor's office to determine what is expected of you financially for the first and subsequent visits.

- Gather and organize your relevant medical records, including blood test results and reports showing diagnoses from other doctors who have treated you for specific conditions, such as orthopedists, cardiologists, hematologists, pulmonologists, dermatologists, internists, surgeons, etc. Many doctors have their own medical records request form, but if yours does not, feel free to use the *Medical Records Release Form* download that I provide to my readers (see the download link on page 153). Or, you can simply make a list of the doctors who have treated or are treating you so that the doctor who needs to review the records can request your medical records for you, as appropriate. (Use the blank *My List of Doctors* form on page 27 to help with this.)

- Fill out the *My Medical Summary* section, beginning on page 21. This section will help the doctor see your brief history at a glance, before he or she reads through each page of your medical records. It will also help you have something to refer to when discussing your medical condition(s).

- Begin filling out a blank *Doctor Visit Details & Journal* page, which starts on page 31. Fill in all your questions for the doctor, organizing them in order of priority. (The remaining portions will be filled out both during and after your appointment.)

- If you are apprehensive about the appointment, ask a family member or trusted friend to accompany you.

- Three days prior to your appointment, confirm the date and time with the doctor's office. Sometimes their office staff will give you a reminder call, but not always.

- Pack the following items to take with you to your in-person appointment:
  - Your referral and filled-out paperwork from the doctor's office (for an initial visit).
  - This book with a bookmark or clip on the corresponding *Doctor Visit Details & Journal* page that you partially filled out with your questions and other information.
  - Your identification card (driver's license or other picture ID).
  - Your health insurance card(s).

On the Day of the Appointment

- Arrive 15 minutes before your in-person appointment, or check-in 10 minutes before your online appointment, just to give yourself time to relax before meeting with your doctor.

- Calm your nerves by going over your paperwork and the pertinent pages in this book to refresh your memory about what you plan to ask and discuss.

During Your Visit

- Introduce yourself and make eye contact. Remember, if you're a new patient, it's important to establish yourself as someone who is interested in fully participating in and taking ownership of your own health.

- If applicable, inform the doctor that you have brought your detailed medical records or refer the doctor to the *My Medical Summary* on page 21 for their review. If the doctor wants a copy, allow the staff to make them. *Never* give away your original medical records.

- Tell the doctor that you have questions and inquire as to the best time to ask them.

- Listen to what the doctor has to say and the answers to your questions. Take notes on your pre-filled out *Doctor Visit Details & Journal* page in this book.

- Keep in mind that first appointments are given more time than appointments for established patients. Either way, the doctor's time is very valuable. Try to be succinct, remembering that the time will go by very quickly.

- When the appointment is about to conclude, be sure to thank your doctor.

After Your Appointment

- If directed by the doctor, make your follow-up appointment with the office staff before you leave. *Always* get an appointment card as a reminder of your next appointment. Yes, even in this day and age of electronic calendars on smart phones and tablets, it is best to always ask for an appointment card just in case you somehow enter the wrong date or time, or some other strange mishap occurs with your electronic calendar. Doctor appointments are too important to allow an error in scheduling. Sometimes, it takes months to get back on their schedule if you accidently miss an appointment.

- Ask the office staff if there is any additional paperwork required for future appointments.

Getting organized and prepared before your appointment will go a long way in helping both you and your doctor get the most out of your visit. It will also help you begin and maintain a good working relationship with your doctor. The next section provides a list of tips for a productive doctor-patient relationship.

The good physician treats the disease; the great physician treats the patient who has the disease.

SIR WILLIAM OSLER

Tips for a Productive Doctor-Patient Relationship

The best relationships in life are based on, among other things, mutual respect and realistic expectations. The relationship you have with your doctor is no different. Be it your family doctor, internist, or a specialist you're seeing for a specific condition, your relationship with your doctor is an important aspect of your medical treatment and healing.

If you don't feel respected or listened to, you'll have a difficult time trusting your doctor. Likewise, if you don't show your doctor that you respect his or her time, or you don't actively participate in your own medical care, your doctor will have a hard time treating you.

To develop the most productive relationship with your doctor, here are a few tips about what to expect from your doctor and what your doctor expects from you:

What You Should Expect from Your Doctor
You should expect your doctor to:

- Listen to you.
- Show you respect.
- Make decisions with you, not for you.
- Be dependable and return your phone calls within 24 to 48 hours.
- Not always have all the answers.
- Value your time.
- Explain anything that you don't understand. Always ask questions if something is not clear.
- Always inform you about your test results and updates to your medical records.
- Encourage and support you and your medical goals.
- Be clear about next steps in scheduling, treatment, costs, etc.
- Understand and help you with getting a second opinion, if you ask for one. Second opinions are usually paid for by insurance.

What Your Doctor Expects from You
Your doctor expects you to:

- Be honest and truthful about your symptoms and changes in your health and updates to your medical records.

- Value their time.
- Ask for clarification if you don't understand something that they are talking about.
- Contact them, if you have not yet heard from the office about your test results in a reasonable amount of time.
- Listen to what they have to say.
- Show them respect and courtesy.
- Share information about any stress you're enduring. Stress often impacts health in ways patients do not fully understand. The more your doctor knows about your mental health, the better he or she can treat you.
- Be open with them if you decide you want a second opinion. Most doctors are happy to help you with getting one. If not, then that doctor is not showing you the respect you deserve.

With these expectations in mind, you will be more comfortable and more equipped to communicate well with your doctor.

Part II

Summarize Your Medical History

A doctor who cannot take a good history,
and a patient who cannot give one,
are in danger of giving and receiving bad treatment.

ANONYMOUS

My Medical Summary

MY CONTACT INFORMATION

NAME:	
ADDRESS:	
CITY, STATE, ZIP:	
TEL: EMAIL:	
EMERGENCY CONTACT:	TEL:

MY MEDICAL DIAGNOSES

DATE OF DIAGNOSIS	NAME OF DIAGNOSIS	DIAGNOSING DOCTOR

MY CHRONIC CONDITIONS & SYMPTOMS

DESCRIPTION OF CHRONIC CONDITION OR SYMPTOM	DATE OF ONSET

My Medical Summary

(CONTINUED)

MY CURRENT MEDICATIONS

NAME OF MEDICATION	DOSAGE	FREQUENCY	REASON	PRESCRIBING DOCTOR	START DATE

MY CURRENT VITAMINS & SUPPLEMENTS

NAME OF VITAMIN OR SUPPLEMENT	DOSAGE	FREQUENCY

My Medical Summary

(CONTINUED)

MY PAST SURGERIES

TYPE OF SURGERY	DATE	HOSPITAL NAME	DOCTOR NAME

MY PAST HOSPITALIZATIONS & ER VISITS

REASON FOR HOSPITALIZATION/ER VISIT	HOSPITAL NAME	DATE(S)

My Medical Summary

(CONTINUED)

MY ALLERGIES

ALLERGEN (MEDICATION, FOOD, OR OTHER)	REACTION(S)	DATE OF ONSET

MY MEDICAL SUMMARY NOTES

_____

_____

_____

_____

_____

_____

_____

_____

_____

_____

My Medical Summary
(CONTINUED)

MY MEDICAL SUMMARY NOTES

_____

_____

_____

_____

_____

_____

_____

_____

_____

_____

_____

_____

_____

_____

_____

_____

_____

_____

_____

_____

_____

My Medical Summary

(CONTINUED)

MY MEDICAL SUMMARY NOTES

My List of Doctors

NAME OF DOCTOR	TYPE OF DOCTOR	ADDRESS	TELEPHONE

My List of Doctors

NAME OF DOCTOR	TYPE OF DOCTOR	ADDRESS	TELEPHONE

PART III

Record Your Doctor Visit Details

*Each patient ought to feel
somewhat the better after the physician's visit,
irrespective of the nature of the illness.*

WARFIELD THEOBALD LONGCOPE

Table of Doctor Appointment Dates

(FOR QUICK REFERENCE TO THE CORRESPONDING
MY DOCTOR VISIT DETAILS & JOURNAL PAGES)

DATE OF DOCTOR VISIT	NAME OF DOCTOR	PAGE
/ /		31
/ /		35
/ /		39
/ /		43
/ /		47
/ /		51
/ /		55
/ /		59
/ /		63
/ /		67
/ /		71
/ /		75
/ /		79
/ /		83
/ /		87

Table of Doctor Appointment Dates

(FOR QUICK REFERENCE TO THE CORRESPONDING
MY DOCTOR VISIT DETAILS & JOURNAL PAGES)

DATE OF DOCTOR VISIT	NAME OF DOCTOR	PAGE
/ /		91
/ /		95
/ /		99
/ /		103
/ /		107
/ /		111
/ /		115
/ /		119
/ /		123
/ /		127
/ /		131
/ /		135
/ /		139
/ /		143
/ /		147

My Doctor Visit Details & Journal

NAME OF DOCTOR / PRACTITIONER: _____

MEDICAL SPECIALTY: _____ APPOINTMENT DATE & TIME: _____

REASON FOR VISIT: O FOLLOW UP   O INITIAL CONSULT   O OTHER _____

VITAL SIGNS: BP _____   PULSE / HR _____   TEMP _____   WEIGHT _____

TODAY'S SYMPTOMS / CONCERNS

_____

_____

LIST OF QUESTIONS TO ASK / TOPICS TO DISCUSS

QUESTION / TOPIC #1:

_____

_____

_____

ANSWER TO #1:

_____

_____

_____

QUESTION / TOPIC #2:

_____

_____

ANSWER TO #2:

_____

_____

_____

My Doctor Visit Details & Journal

APPOINTMENT DATE: ___/___/___ *(CONTINUED)*

QUESTION / TOPIC #3:

ANSWER TO #3:

QUESTION / TOPIC #4:

ANSWER TO #4:

QUESTION / TOPIC #5:

ANSWER TO #5:

My Doctor Visit Details & Journal

APPOINTMENT DATE: ___/___/___ (CONTINUED)

DOCTOR'S / PRACTITIONER'S INSTRUCTIONS, DIAGNOSIS & ACTION PLAN FOR ME

FOLLOW-UP APPOINTMENT DATE & TIME:

NEW MEDICATION(S):

FOLLOW-UP LAB TESTS:

FOLLOW-UP IMAGING:

MY REMINDERS / THOUGHTS / NOTES

My Doctor Visit Details & Journal

APPOINTMENT DATE: ___/___/___ *(CONTINUED)*

MY REMINDERS / THOUGHTS / NOTES

_____

_____

_____

_____

_____

_____

_____

_____

_____

_____

_____

_____

_____

_____

_____

_____

_____

_____

_____

_____

_____

My Doctor Visit Details & Journal

NAME OF DOCTOR / PRACTITIONER: _____

MEDICAL SPECIALTY: _____ APPOINTMENT DATE & TIME: _____

REASON FOR VISIT: ○ FOLLOW UP   ○ INITIAL CONSULT   ○ OTHER _____

VITAL SIGNS: BP _____ PULSE / HR _____ TEMP _____ WEIGHT _____

TODAY'S SYMPTOMS / CONCERNS

_____

_____

LIST OF QUESTIONS TO ASK / TOPICS TO DISCUSS

QUESTION / TOPIC #1:

_____

_____

ANSWER TO #1:

_____

_____

_____

QUESTION / TOPIC #2:

_____

_____

ANSWER TO #2:

_____

_____

_____

My Doctor Visit Details & Journal

APPOINTMENT DATE: ___/___/___ (*CONTINUED*)

QUESTION / TOPIC #3:

_____

_____

ANSWER TO #3:

_____

_____

QUESTION / TOPIC #4:

_____

_____

ANSWER TO #4:

_____

_____

QUESTION / TOPIC #5:

_____

_____

ANSWER TO #5:

_____

_____

My Doctor Visit Details & Journal

APPOINTMENT DATE: ___/___/___ (CONTINUED)

DOCTOR'S / PRACTITIONER'S INSTRUCTIONS, DIAGNOSIS & ACTION PLAN FOR ME

FOLLOW-UP APPOINTMENT DATE & TIME:

NEW MEDICATION(S):

FOLLOW-UP LAB TESTS:

FOLLOW-UP IMAGING:

MY REMINDERS / THOUGHTS / NOTES

My Doctor Visit Details & Journal

APPOINTMENT DATE: ___/___/___ (*CONTINUED*)

MY REMINDERS / THOUGHTS / NOTES

_____

_____

_____

_____

_____

_____

_____

_____

_____

_____

_____

_____

_____

_____

_____

_____

_____

_____

_____

_____

_____

My Doctor Visit Details & Journal

NAME OF DOCTOR / PRACTITIONER: _____

MEDICAL SPECIALTY: _____ APPOINTMENT DATE & TIME: _____

REASON FOR VISIT: O FOLLOW UP   O INITIAL CONSULT   O OTHER _____

VITAL SIGNS: BP _____   PULSE / HR _____   TEMP _____   WEIGHT _____

TODAY'S SYMPTOMS / CONCERNS

_____

_____

LIST OF QUESTIONS TO ASK / TOPICS TO DISCUSS

QUESTION / TOPIC #1:

_____

_____

_____

ANSWER TO #1:

_____

_____

_____

QUESTION / TOPIC #2:

_____

_____

ANSWER TO #2:

_____

_____

_____

My Doctor Visit Details & Journal

APPOINTMENT DATE: ___/___/___ (*CONTINUED*)

QUESTION / TOPIC #3:

ANSWER TO #3:

QUESTION / TOPIC #4:

ANSWER TO #4:

QUESTION / TOPIC #5:

ANSWER TO #5:

My Doctor Visit Details & Journal

APPOINTMENT DATE: ___/___/___ (CONTINUED)

DOCTOR'S / PRACTITIONER'S INSTRUCTIONS, DIAGNOSIS & ACTION PLAN FOR ME

FOLLOW-UP APPOINTMENT DATE & TIME:

NEW MEDICATION(S):

FOLLOW-UP LAB TESTS:

FOLLOW-UP IMAGING:

MY REMINDERS / THOUGHTS / NOTES

My Doctor Visit Details & Journal

APPOINTMENT DATE: ___/___/___ (*CONTINUED*)

MY REMINDERS / THOUGHTS / NOTES

My Doctor Visit Details & Journal

NAME OF DOCTOR / PRACTITIONER: _____

MEDICAL SPECIALTY: _____ APPOINTMENT DATE & TIME: _____

REASON FOR VISIT: ○ FOLLOW UP   ○ INITIAL CONSULT   ○ OTHER _____

VITAL SIGNS: BP _____   PULSE / HR _____   TEMP _____   WEIGHT _____

TODAY'S SYMPTOMS / CONCERNS

_____

_____

LIST OF QUESTIONS TO ASK / TOPICS TO DISCUSS

QUESTION / TOPIC #1:

_____

_____

_____

ANSWER TO #1:

_____

_____

QUESTION / TOPIC #2:

_____

_____

ANSWER TO #2:

_____

_____

My Doctor Visit Details & Journal

QUESTION / TOPIC #3:

_____

_____

_____

ANSWER TO #3:

_____

_____

_____

QUESTION / TOPIC #4:

_____

_____

ANSWER TO #4:

_____

_____

_____

QUESTION / TOPIC #5:

_____

_____

ANSWER TO #5:

_____

_____

_____

My Doctor Visit Details & Journal

APPOINTMENT DATE: ___/___/___ (CONTINUED)

DOCTOR'S / PRACTITIONER'S INSTRUCTIONS, DIAGNOSIS & ACTION PLAN FOR ME

FOLLOW-UP APPOINTMENT DATE & TIME:

NEW MEDICATION(S):

FOLLOW-UP LAB TESTS:

FOLLOW-UP IMAGING:

MY REMINDERS / THOUGHTS / NOTES

My Doctor Visit Details & Journal

APPOINTMENT DATE: ___/___/___ *(CONTINUED)*

MY REMINDERS / THOUGHTS / NOTES

_____

_____

_____

_____

_____

_____

_____

_____

_____

_____

_____

_____

_____

_____

_____

_____

_____

_____

_____

_____

_____

_____

My Doctor Visit Details & Journal

NAME OF DOCTOR / PRACTITIONER: _____

MEDICAL SPECIALTY: _____ APPOINTMENT DATE & TIME: _____

REASON FOR VISIT: ○ FOLLOW UP ○ INITIAL CONSULT ○ OTHER _____

VITAL SIGNS: BP _____ PULSE / HR _____ TEMP _____ WEIGHT _____

TODAY'S SYMPTOMS / CONCERNS

_____

_____

LIST OF QUESTIONS TO ASK / TOPICS TO DISCUSS

QUESTION / TOPIC #1:

_____

_____

_____

ANSWER TO #1:

_____

_____

QUESTION / TOPIC #2:

_____

_____

ANSWER TO #2:

_____

_____

My Doctor Visit Details & Journal

APPOINTMENT DATE: ___/___/___ *(CONTINUED)*

QUESTION / TOPIC #3:

_____
_____
_____

ANSWER TO #3:

_____
_____
_____

QUESTION / TOPIC #4:

_____
_____
_____

ANSWER TO #4:

_____
_____
_____

QUESTION / TOPIC #5:

_____
_____
_____

ANSWER TO #5:

_____
_____
_____

My Doctor Visit Details & Journal

APPOINTMENT DATE: ___/___/___ (CONTINUED)

DOCTOR'S / PRACTITIONER'S INSTRUCTIONS, DIAGNOSIS & ACTION PLAN FOR ME

FOLLOW-UP APPOINTMENT DATE & TIME:

NEW MEDICATION(S):

FOLLOW-UP LAB TESTS:

FOLLOW-UP IMAGING:

MY REMINDERS / THOUGHTS / NOTES

My Doctor Visit Details & Journal

APPOINTMENT DATE: ___/___/___ (*CONTINUED*)

MY REMINDERS / THOUGHTS / NOTES

My Doctor Visit Details & Journal

NAME OF DOCTOR / PRACTITIONER: _____

MEDICAL SPECIALTY: _____ APPOINTMENT DATE & TIME: _____

REASON FOR VISIT: ○ FOLLOW UP   ○ INITIAL CONSULT   ○ OTHER _____

VITAL SIGNS: BP _____   PULSE / HR _____   TEMP _____   WEIGHT _____

TODAY'S SYMPTOMS / CONCERNS

_____

_____

LIST OF QUESTIONS TO ASK / TOPICS TO DISCUSS

QUESTION / TOPIC #1:

_____

_____

ANSWER TO #1:

_____

_____

QUESTION / TOPIC #2:

_____

_____

ANSWER TO #2:

_____

_____

My Doctor Visit Details & Journal

APPOINTMENT DATE: ___/___/___ (*CONTINUED*)

QUESTION / TOPIC #3:

ANSWER TO #3:

QUESTION / TOPIC #4:

ANSWER TO #4:

QUESTION / TOPIC #5:

ANSWER TO #5:

My Doctor Visit Details & Journal

APPOINTMENT DATE: ___/___/___ (*CONTINUED*)

DOCTOR'S / PRACTITIONER'S INSTRUCTIONS, DIAGNOSIS & ACTION PLAN FOR ME

FOLLOW-UP APPOINTMENT DATE & TIME:

NEW MEDICATION(S):

FOLLOW-UP LAB TESTS:

FOLLOW-UP IMAGING:

MY REMINDERS / THOUGHTS / NOTES

My Doctor Visit Details & Journal

APPOINTMENT DATE: ___/___/___ (CONTINUED)

MY REMINDERS / THOUGHTS / NOTES

My Doctor Visit Details & Journal

NAME OF DOCTOR / PRACTITIONER: _____

MEDICAL SPECIALTY: _____ APPOINTMENT DATE & TIME: _____

REASON FOR VISIT: ○ FOLLOW UP ○ INITIAL CONSULT ○ OTHER _____

VITAL SIGNS: BP _____ PULSE / HR _____ TEMP _____ WEIGHT _____

TODAY'S SYMPTOMS / CONCERNS

_____

_____

LIST OF QUESTIONS TO ASK / TOPICS TO DISCUSS

QUESTION / TOPIC #1:

_____

_____

ANSWER TO #1:

_____

_____

_____

QUESTION / TOPIC #2:

_____

_____

ANSWER TO #2:

_____

_____

_____

My Doctor Visit Details & Journal

APPOINTMENT DATE: ___/___/___ *(CONTINUED)*

QUESTION / TOPIC #3:

_____

_____

_____

ANSWER TO #3:

_____

_____

_____

QUESTION / TOPIC #4:

_____

_____

_____

ANSWER TO #4:

_____

_____

_____

QUESTION / TOPIC #5:

_____

_____

_____

ANSWER TO #5:

_____

_____

_____

My Doctor Visit Details & Journal

DOCTOR'S / PRACTITIONER'S INSTRUCTIONS, DIAGNOSIS & ACTION PLAN FOR ME

FOLLOW-UP APPOINTMENT DATE & TIME:

NEW MEDICATION(S):

FOLLOW-UP LAB TESTS:

FOLLOW-UP IMAGING:

MY REMINDERS / THOUGHTS / NOTES

My Doctor Visit Details & Journal

APPOINTMENT DATE: ___/___/___ (CONTINUED)

MY REMINDERS / THOUGHTS / NOTES

My Doctor Visit Details & Journal

NAME OF DOCTOR / PRACTITIONER: _____

MEDICAL SPECIALTY: _____ APPOINTMENT DATE & TIME: _____

REASON FOR VISIT: O FOLLOW UP   O INITIAL CONSULT   O OTHER _____

VITAL SIGNS: BP _____   PULSE / HR _____   TEMP _____   WEIGHT _____

TODAY'S SYMPTOMS / CONCERNS

_____

_____

LIST OF QUESTIONS TO ASK / TOPICS TO DISCUSS

QUESTION / TOPIC #1:

_____

_____

_____

ANSWER TO #1:

_____

_____

QUESTION / TOPIC #2:

_____

_____

ANSWER TO #2:

_____

_____

My Doctor Visit Details & Journal

APPOINTMENT DATE: ___/___/___ (*CONTINUED*)

QUESTION / TOPIC #3:

_____

_____

_____

ANSWER TO #3:

_____

_____

_____

QUESTION / TOPIC #4:

_____

_____

_____

ANSWER TO #4:

_____

_____

_____

QUESTION / TOPIC #5:

_____

_____

_____

ANSWER TO #5:

_____

_____

_____

My Doctor Visit Details & Journal

APPOINTMENT DATE: ___/___/___ (CONTINUED)

DOCTOR'S / PRACTITIONER'S INSTRUCTIONS, DIAGNOSIS & ACTION PLAN FOR ME

FOLLOW-UP APPOINTMENT DATE & TIME:

NEW MEDICATION(S):

FOLLOW-UP LAB TESTS:

FOLLOW-UP IMAGING:

MY REMINDERS / THOUGHTS / NOTES

My Doctor Visit Details & Journal

APPOINTMENT DATE: ___/___/___ (*CONTINUED*)

MY REMINDERS / THOUGHTS / NOTES

My Doctor Visit Details & Journal

NAME OF DOCTOR / PRACTITIONER: _____

MEDICAL SPECIALTY: _____ APPOINTMENT DATE & TIME:_____

REASON FOR VISIT: O FOLLOW UP   O INITIAL CONSULT   O OTHER _____

VITAL SIGNS: BP_____   PULSE / HR _____   TEMP _____   WEIGHT _____

TODAY'S SYMPTOMS / CONCERNS

_____

_____

LIST OF QUESTIONS TO ASK / TOPICS TO DISCUSS

QUESTION / TOPIC #1:

_____

_____

_____

ANSWER TO #1:

_____

_____

QUESTION / TOPIC #2:

_____

_____

ANSWER TO #2:

_____

_____

My Doctor Visit Details & Journal

APPOINTMENT DATE: ___/___/___ (*CONTINUED*)

QUESTION / TOPIC #3:

ANSWER TO #3:

QUESTION / TOPIC #4:

ANSWER TO #4:

QUESTION / TOPIC #5:

ANSWER TO #5:

My Doctor Visit Details & Journal

APPOINTMENT DATE: ___/___/___ (CONTINUED)

DOCTOR'S / PRACTITIONER'S INSTRUCTIONS, DIAGNOSIS & ACTION PLAN FOR ME

FOLLOW-UP APPOINTMENT DATE & TIME:

NEW MEDICATION(S):

FOLLOW-UP LAB TESTS:

FOLLOW-UP IMAGING:

MY REMINDERS / THOUGHTS / NOTES

My Doctor Visit Details & Journal

APPOINTMENT DATE: ___/___/___ (*CONTINUED*)

MY REMINDERS / THOUGHTS / NOTES

My Doctor Visit Details & Journal

NAME OF DOCTOR / PRACTITIONER: _____

MEDICAL SPECIALTY: _____ APPOINTMENT DATE & TIME: _____

REASON FOR VISIT: ○ FOLLOW UP   ○ INITIAL CONSULT   ○ OTHER _____

VITAL SIGNS: BP _____   PULSE / HR _____   TEMP _____   WEIGHT _____

TODAY'S SYMPTOMS / CONCERNS

_____

_____

LIST OF QUESTIONS TO ASK / TOPICS TO DISCUSS

QUESTION / TOPIC #1:

_____

_____

_____

ANSWER TO #1:

_____

_____

QUESTION / TOPIC #2:

_____

_____

ANSWER TO #2:

_____

_____

My Doctor Visit Details & Journal

APPOINTMENT DATE: ___/___/___ *(CONTINUED)*

QUESTION / TOPIC #3:

_____

_____

_____

ANSWER TO #3:

_____

_____

_____

QUESTION / TOPIC #4:

_____

_____

ANSWER TO #4:

_____

_____

_____

QUESTION / TOPIC #5:

_____

_____

ANSWER TO #5:

_____

_____

_____

My Doctor Visit Details & Journal

APPOINTMENT DATE: ___/___/___ (*CONTINUED*)

DOCTOR'S / PRACTITIONER'S INSTRUCTIONS, DIAGNOSIS & ACTION PLAN FOR ME

FOLLOW-UP APPOINTMENT DATE & TIME:

NEW MEDICATION(S):

FOLLOW-UP LAB TESTS:

FOLLOW-UP IMAGING:

MY REMINDERS / THOUGHTS / NOTES

My Doctor Visit Details & Journal

APPOINTMENT DATE: ___/___/___ (CONTINUED)

MY REMINDERS / THOUGHTS / NOTES

My Doctor Visit Details & Journal

NAME OF DOCTOR / PRACTITIONER: _____

MEDICAL SPECIALTY: _____ APPOINTMENT DATE & TIME: _____

REASON FOR VISIT: ○ FOLLOW UP   ○ INITIAL CONSULT   ○ OTHER _____

VITAL SIGNS: BP _____   PULSE / HR _____   TEMP _____   WEIGHT _____

TODAY'S SYMPTOMS / CONCERNS

_____

_____

LIST OF QUESTIONS TO ASK / TOPICS TO DISCUSS

QUESTION / TOPIC #1:

_____

_____

_____

ANSWER TO #1:

_____

_____

_____

QUESTION / TOPIC #2:

_____

_____

ANSWER TO #2:

_____

_____

_____

My Doctor Visit Details & Journal

APPOINTMENT DATE: ___/___/___ (CONTINUED)

QUESTION / TOPIC #3:

_____

_____

_____

ANSWER TO #3:

_____

_____

_____

QUESTION / TOPIC #4:

_____

_____

_____

ANSWER TO #4:

_____

_____

_____

QUESTION / TOPIC #5:

_____

_____

_____

ANSWER TO #5:

_____

_____

_____

My Doctor Visit Details & Journal

APPOINTMENT DATE: ___/___/___ (CONTINUED)

DOCTOR'S / PRACTITIONER'S INSTRUCTIONS, DIAGNOSIS & ACTION PLAN FOR ME

FOLLOW-UP APPOINTMENT DATE & TIME:

NEW MEDICATION(S):

FOLLOW-UP LAB TESTS:

FOLLOW-UP IMAGING:

MY REMINDERS / THOUGHTS / NOTES

My Doctor Visit Details & Journal

APPOINTMENT DATE: ___/___/___ (*CONTINUED*)

MY REMINDERS / THOUGHTS / NOTES

My Doctor Visit Details & Journal

NAME OF DOCTOR / PRACTITIONER: _____

MEDICAL SPECIALTY: _____ APPOINTMENT DATE & TIME: _____

REASON FOR VISIT: ○ FOLLOW UP   ○ INITIAL CONSULT   ○ OTHER _____

VITAL SIGNS: BP _____   PULSE / HR _____   TEMP _____   WEIGHT _____

TODAY'S SYMPTOMS / CONCERNS

_____

_____

LIST OF QUESTIONS TO ASK / TOPICS TO DISCUSS

QUESTION / TOPIC #1:

_____

_____

_____

ANSWER TO #1:

_____

_____

QUESTION / TOPIC #2:

_____

_____

ANSWER TO #2:

_____

_____

My Doctor Visit Details & Journal

APPOINTMENT DATE: ___/___/___ (CONTINUED)

QUESTION / TOPIC #3:

ANSWER TO #3:

QUESTION / TOPIC #4:

ANSWER TO #4:

QUESTION / TOPIC #5:

ANSWER TO #5:

My Doctor Visit Details & Journal

APPOINTMENT DATE: ___/___/___ (*CONTINUED*)

DOCTOR'S / PRACTITIONER'S INSTRUCTIONS, DIAGNOSIS & ACTION PLAN FOR ME

FOLLOW-UP APPOINTMENT DATE & TIME:

NEW MEDICATION(S):

FOLLOW-UP LAB TESTS:

FOLLOW-UP IMAGING:

MY REMINDERS / THOUGHTS / NOTES

My Doctor Visit Details & Journal

APPOINTMENT DATE: ___/___/___ (CONTINUED)

MY REMINDERS / THOUGHTS / NOTES

My Doctor Visit Details & Journal

NAME OF DOCTOR / PRACTITIONER: _____

MEDICAL SPECIALTY: _____ APPOINTMENT DATE & TIME: _____

REASON FOR VISIT: ○ FOLLOW UP ○ INITIAL CONSULT ○ OTHER _____

VITAL SIGNS: BP _____ PULSE / HR _____ TEMP _____ WEIGHT _____

TODAY'S SYMPTOMS / CONCERNS

_____

_____

LIST OF QUESTIONS TO ASK / TOPICS TO DISCUSS

QUESTION / TOPIC #1:

_____

_____

_____

ANSWER TO #1:

_____

_____

_____

QUESTION / TOPIC #2:

_____

_____

ANSWER TO #2:

_____

_____

_____

My Doctor Visit Details & Journal

APPOINTMENT DATE: ___/___/___ (CONTINUED)

QUESTION / TOPIC #3:

ANSWER TO #3:

QUESTION / TOPIC #4:

ANSWER TO #4:

QUESTION / TOPIC #5:

ANSWER TO #5:

My Doctor Visit Details & Journal

APPOINTMENT DATE: ___/___/___ (CONTINUED)

DOCTOR'S / PRACTITIONER'S INSTRUCTIONS, DIAGNOSIS & ACTION PLAN FOR ME

FOLLOW-UP APPOINTMENT DATE & TIME:

NEW MEDICATION(S):

FOLLOW-UP LAB TESTS:

FOLLOW-UP IMAGING:

MY REMINDERS / THOUGHTS / NOTES

My Doctor Visit Details & Journal

APPOINTMENT DATE: ___/___/___ (*CONTINUED*)

MY REMINDERS / THOUGHTS / NOTES

My Doctor Visit Details & Journal

NAME OF DOCTOR / PRACTITIONER: _____

MEDICAL SPECIALTY: _____ APPOINTMENT DATE & TIME: _____

REASON FOR VISIT: ○ FOLLOW UP   ○ INITIAL CONSULT   ○ OTHER _____

VITAL SIGNS: BP _____ PULSE / HR _____ TEMP _____ WEIGHT _____

TODAY'S SYMPTOMS / CONCERNS

_____

_____

LIST OF QUESTIONS TO ASK / TOPICS TO DISCUSS

QUESTION / TOPIC #1:

_____

_____

_____

ANSWER TO #1:

_____

_____

_____

QUESTION / TOPIC #2:

_____

_____

ANSWER TO #2:

_____

_____

_____

My Doctor Visit Details & Journal

APPOINTMENT DATE: ___/___/___ (CONTINUED)

QUESTION / TOPIC #3:

ANSWER TO #3:

QUESTION / TOPIC #4:

ANSWER TO #4:

QUESTION / TOPIC #5:

ANSWER TO #5:

My Doctor Visit Details & Journal

APPOINTMENT DATE: ___/___/___ (CONTINUED)

DOCTOR'S / PRACTITIONER'S INSTRUCTIONS, DIAGNOSIS & ACTION PLAN FOR ME

FOLLOW-UP APPOINTMENT DATE & TIME:

NEW MEDICATION(S):

FOLLOW-UP LAB TESTS:

FOLLOW-UP IMAGING:

MY REMINDERS / THOUGHTS / NOTES

My Doctor Visit Details & Journal

APPOINTMENT DATE: ___/___/___ (*CONTINUED*)

MY REMINDERS / THOUGHTS / NOTES

_____

_____

_____

_____

_____

_____

_____

_____

_____

_____

_____

_____

_____

_____

_____

_____

_____

_____

_____

_____

_____

My Doctor Visit Details & Journal

NAME OF DOCTOR / PRACTITIONER: _____

MEDICAL SPECIALTY: _____ APPOINTMENT DATE & TIME: _____

REASON FOR VISIT: ○ FOLLOW UP ○ INITIAL CONSULT ○ OTHER _____

VITAL SIGNS: BP _____ PULSE / HR _____ TEMP _____ WEIGHT _____

TODAY'S SYMPTOMS / CONCERNS

_____

_____

LIST OF QUESTIONS TO ASK / TOPICS TO DISCUSS

QUESTION / TOPIC #1:

_____

_____

_____

ANSWER TO #1:

_____

_____

_____

QUESTION / TOPIC #2:

_____

_____

ANSWER TO #2:

_____

_____

_____

My Doctor Visit Details & Journal

APPOINTMENT DATE: ___/___/___ *(CONTINUED)*

QUESTION / TOPIC #3:

ANSWER TO #3:

QUESTION / TOPIC #4:

ANSWER TO #4:

QUESTION / TOPIC #5:

ANSWER TO #5:

My Doctor Visit Details & Journal

APPOINTMENT DATE: ___/___/___ (*CONTINUED*)

DOCTOR'S / PRACTITIONER'S INSTRUCTIONS, DIAGNOSIS & ACTION PLAN FOR ME

FOLLOW-UP APPOINTMENT DATE & TIME:

NEW MEDICATION(S):

FOLLOW-UP LAB TESTS:

FOLLOW-UP IMAGING:

MY REMINDERS / THOUGHTS / NOTES

My Doctor Visit Details & Journal

APPOINTMENT DATE: ___/___/___ (*CONTINUED*)

MY REMINDERS / THOUGHTS / NOTES

My Doctor Visit Details & Journal

NAME OF DOCTOR / PRACTITIONER: _____

MEDICAL SPECIALTY: _____ APPOINTMENT DATE & TIME: _____

REASON FOR VISIT: O FOLLOW UP   O INITIAL CONSULT   O OTHER _____

VITAL SIGNS: BP _____   PULSE / HR _____   TEMP _____   WEIGHT _____

TODAY'S SYMPTOMS / CONCERNS

_____

_____

LIST OF QUESTIONS TO ASK / TOPICS TO DISCUSS

QUESTION / TOPIC #1:

_____

_____

_____

ANSWER TO #1:

_____

_____

_____

QUESTION / TOPIC #2:

_____

_____

ANSWER TO #2:

_____

_____

_____

My Doctor Visit Details & Journal

APPOINTMENT DATE: ___/ ___/ ___ (*CONTINUED*)

QUESTION / TOPIC #3:

ANSWER TO #3:

QUESTION / TOPIC #4:

ANSWER TO #4:

QUESTION / TOPIC #5:

ANSWER TO #5:

My Doctor Visit Details & Journal

APPOINTMENT DATE: ___/___/___ (CONTINUED)

DOCTOR'S / PRACTITIONER'S INSTRUCTIONS, DIAGNOSIS & ACTION PLAN FOR ME

FOLLOW-UP APPOINTMENT DATE & TIME:

NEW MEDICATION(S):

FOLLOW-UP LAB TESTS:

FOLLOW-UP IMAGING:

MY REMINDERS / THOUGHTS / NOTES

My Doctor Visit Details & Journal

APPOINTMENT DATE: ___/___/___ *(CONTINUED)*

MY REMINDERS / THOUGHTS / NOTES

My Doctor Visit Details & Journal

NAME OF DOCTOR / PRACTITIONER: _____

MEDICAL SPECIALTY: _____ APPOINTMENT DATE & TIME: _____

REASON FOR VISIT: ○ FOLLOW UP ○ INITIAL CONSULT ○ OTHER _____

VITAL SIGNS: BP _____ PULSE / HR _____ TEMP _____ WEIGHT _____

TODAY'S SYMPTOMS / CONCERNS

_____

_____

LIST OF QUESTIONS TO ASK / TOPICS TO DISCUSS

QUESTION / TOPIC #1:

_____

_____

_____

ANSWER TO #1:

_____

_____

_____

QUESTION / TOPIC #2:

_____

_____

ANSWER TO #2:

_____

_____

_____

My Doctor Visit Details & Journal

APPOINTMENT DATE: ___/___/___ (*CONTINUED*)

QUESTION / TOPIC #3:

_____

_____

_____

ANSWER TO #3:

_____

_____

_____

QUESTION / TOPIC #4:

_____

_____

_____

ANSWER TO #4:

_____

_____

_____

QUESTION / TOPIC #5:

_____

_____

_____

ANSWER TO #5:

_____

_____

_____

My Doctor Visit Details & Journal

APPOINTMENT DATE: ___/___/___ (CONTINUED)

DOCTOR'S / PRACTITIONER'S INSTRUCTIONS, DIAGNOSIS & ACTION PLAN FOR ME

FOLLOW-UP APPOINTMENT DATE & TIME:

NEW MEDICATION(S):

FOLLOW-UP LAB TESTS:

FOLLOW-UP IMAGING:

MY REMINDERS / THOUGHTS / NOTES

My Doctor Visit Details & Journal

APPOINTMENT DATE: ___/___/___ (*CONTINUED*)

MY REMINDERS / THOUGHTS / NOTES

My Doctor Visit Details & Journal

NAME OF DOCTOR / PRACTITIONER: _____

MEDICAL SPECIALTY: _____ APPOINTMENT DATE & TIME: _____

REASON FOR VISIT: ○ FOLLOW UP   ○ INITIAL CONSULT   ○ OTHER _____

VITAL SIGNS: BP _____   PULSE / HR _____   TEMP _____   WEIGHT _____

TODAY'S SYMPTOMS / CONCERNS

_____

_____

LIST OF QUESTIONS TO ASK / TOPICS TO DISCUSS

QUESTION / TOPIC #1:

_____

_____

_____

ANSWER TO #1:

_____

_____

_____

QUESTION / TOPIC #2:

_____

_____

ANSWER TO #2:

_____

_____

_____

My Doctor Visit Details & Journal

APPOINTMENT DATE: ___/___/___ *(CONTINUED)*

QUESTION / TOPIC #3:

ANSWER TO #3:

QUESTION / TOPIC #4:

ANSWER TO #4:

QUESTION / TOPIC #5:

ANSWER TO #5:

My Doctor Visit Details & Journal

APPOINTMENT DATE: ___/___/___ (CONTINUED)

DOCTOR'S / PRACTITIONER'S INSTRUCTIONS, DIAGNOSIS & ACTION PLAN FOR ME

FOLLOW-UP APPOINTMENT DATE & TIME:

NEW MEDICATION(S):

FOLLOW-UP LAB TESTS:

FOLLOW-UP IMAGING:

MY REMINDERS / THOUGHTS / NOTES

My Doctor Visit Details & Journal

APPOINTMENT DATE: ____/____/____ (*CONTINUED*)

MY REMINDERS / THOUGHTS / NOTES

My Doctor Visit Details & Journal

NAME OF DOCTOR / PRACTITIONER: _____

MEDICAL SPECIALTY: _____ APPOINTMENT DATE & TIME: _____

REASON FOR VISIT: ○ FOLLOW UP ○ INITIAL CONSULT ○ OTHER _____

VITAL SIGNS: BP _____ PULSE / HR _____ TEMP _____ WEIGHT _____

TODAY'S SYMPTOMS / CONCERNS

_____

_____

LIST OF QUESTIONS TO ASK / TOPICS TO DISCUSS

QUESTION / TOPIC #1:

_____

_____

_____

ANSWER TO #1:

_____

_____

_____

QUESTION / TOPIC #2:

_____

_____

ANSWER TO #2:

_____

_____

_____

My Doctor Visit Details & Journal

APPOINTMENT DATE: ___/___/___ *(CONTINUED)*

QUESTION / TOPIC #3:

ANSWER TO #3:

QUESTION / TOPIC #4:

ANSWER TO #4:

QUESTION / TOPIC #5:

ANSWER TO #5:

My Doctor Visit Details & Journal

APPOINTMENT DATE: ___/___/___ (CONTINUED)

DOCTOR'S / PRACTITIONER'S INSTRUCTIONS, DIAGNOSIS & ACTION PLAN FOR ME

FOLLOW-UP APPOINTMENT DATE & TIME:

NEW MEDICATION(S):

FOLLOW-UP LAB TESTS:

FOLLOW-UP IMAGING:

MY REMINDERS / THOUGHTS / NOTES

My Doctor Visit Details & Journal

APPOINTMENT DATE: ___/___/___ *(CONTINUED)*

MY REMINDERS / THOUGHTS / NOTES

My Doctor Visit Details & Journal

NAME OF DOCTOR / PRACTITIONER: _____

MEDICAL SPECIALTY: _____ APPOINTMENT DATE & TIME: _____

REASON FOR VISIT: ○ FOLLOW UP   ○ INITIAL CONSULT   ○ OTHER _____

VITAL SIGNS: BP _____ PULSE / HR _____ TEMP _____ WEIGHT _____

TODAY'S SYMPTOMS / CONCERNS

_____

_____

LIST OF QUESTIONS TO ASK / TOPICS TO DISCUSS

QUESTION / TOPIC #1:

_____

_____

ANSWER TO #1:

_____

_____

QUESTION / TOPIC #2:

_____

_____

ANSWER TO #2:

_____

_____

My Doctor Visit Details & Journal

QUESTION / TOPIC #3:

_____

_____

_____

ANSWER TO #3:

_____

_____

_____

QUESTION / TOPIC #4:

_____

_____

_____

ANSWER TO #4:

_____

_____

_____

QUESTION / TOPIC #5:

_____

_____

_____

ANSWER TO #5:

_____

_____

_____

My Doctor Visit Details & Journal

APPOINTMENT DATE: ___/___/___ (CONTINUED)

DOCTOR'S / PRACTITIONER'S INSTRUCTIONS, DIAGNOSIS & ACTION PLAN FOR ME

FOLLOW-UP APPOINTMENT DATE & TIME:

NEW MEDICATION(S):

FOLLOW-UP LAB TESTS:

FOLLOW-UP IMAGING:

MY REMINDERS / THOUGHTS / NOTES

My Doctor Visit Details & Journal

APPOINTMENT DATE: ____/____/____ (*CONTINUED*)

MY REMINDERS / THOUGHTS / NOTES

My Doctor Visit Details & Journal

NAME OF DOCTOR / PRACTITIONER: _____

MEDICAL SPECIALTY: _____ APPOINTMENT DATE & TIME: _____

REASON FOR VISIT: ○ FOLLOW UP ○ INITIAL CONSULT ○ OTHER _____

VITAL SIGNS: BP_____ PULSE / HR _____ TEMP _____ WEIGHT _____

TODAY'S SYMPTOMS / CONCERNS

_____

_____

LIST OF QUESTIONS TO ASK / TOPICS TO DISCUSS

QUESTION / TOPIC #1:

_____

_____

_____

ANSWER TO #1:

_____

_____

_____

QUESTION / TOPIC #2:

_____

_____

ANSWER TO #2:

_____

_____

_____

My Doctor Visit Details & Journal

QUESTION / TOPIC #3:

ANSWER TO #3:

QUESTION / TOPIC #4:

ANSWER TO #4:

QUESTION / TOPIC #5:

ANSWER TO #5:

My Doctor Visit Details & Journal

APPOINTMENT DATE: ___/___/___ (CONTINUED)

DOCTOR'S / PRACTITIONER'S INSTRUCTIONS, DIAGNOSIS & ACTION PLAN FOR ME

FOLLOW-UP APPOINTMENT DATE & TIME:

NEW MEDICATION(S):

FOLLOW-UP LAB TESTS:

FOLLOW-UP IMAGING:

MY REMINDERS / THOUGHTS / NOTES

My Doctor Visit Details & Journal

APPOINTMENT DATE: ___/___/___ (*CONTINUED*)

MY REMINDERS / THOUGHTS / NOTES

My Doctor Visit Details & Journal

NAME OF DOCTOR / PRACTITIONER: _____

MEDICAL SPECIALTY: _____ APPOINTMENT DATE & TIME: _____

REASON FOR VISIT: ○ FOLLOW UP ○ INITIAL CONSULT ○ OTHER _____

VITAL SIGNS: BP _____ PULSE / HR _____ TEMP _____ WEIGHT _____

TODAY'S SYMPTOMS / CONCERNS

_____

_____

LIST OF QUESTIONS TO ASK / TOPICS TO DISCUSS

QUESTION / TOPIC #1:

_____

_____

_____

ANSWER TO #1:

_____

_____

_____

QUESTION / TOPIC #2:

_____

_____

ANSWER TO #2:

_____

_____

_____

My Doctor Visit Details & Journal

QUESTION / TOPIC #3:

ANSWER TO #3:

QUESTION / TOPIC #4:

ANSWER TO #4:

QUESTION / TOPIC #5:

ANSWER TO #5:

My Doctor Visit Details & Journal

APPOINTMENT DATE: ___/___/___ (CONTINUED)

DOCTOR'S / PRACTITIONER'S INSTRUCTIONS, DIAGNOSIS & ACTION PLAN FOR ME

FOLLOW-UP APPOINTMENT DATE & TIME:

NEW MEDICATION(S):

FOLLOW-UP LAB TESTS:

FOLLOW-UP IMAGING:

MY REMINDERS / THOUGHTS / NOTES

My Doctor Visit Details & Journal

APPOINTMENT DATE: ___/___/___ (*CONTINUED*)

MY REMINDERS / THOUGHTS / NOTES

My Doctor Visit Details & Journal

NAME OF DOCTOR / PRACTITIONER: _____

MEDICAL SPECIALTY: _____ APPOINTMENT DATE & TIME: _____

REASON FOR VISIT: O FOLLOW UP   O INITIAL CONSULT   O OTHER _____

VITAL SIGNS: BP _____   PULSE / HR _____   TEMP _____   WEIGHT _____

TODAY'S SYMPTOMS / CONCERNS

_____

_____

LIST OF QUESTIONS TO ASK / TOPICS TO DISCUSS

QUESTION / TOPIC #1:

_____

_____

_____

ANSWER TO #1:

_____

_____

QUESTION / TOPIC #2:

_____

_____

ANSWER TO #2:

_____

_____

My Doctor Visit Details & Journal

APPOINTMENT DATE: ___/___/___ (CONTINUED)

QUESTION / TOPIC #3:

ANSWER TO #3:

QUESTION / TOPIC #4:

ANSWER TO #4:

QUESTION / TOPIC #5:

ANSWER TO #5:

My Doctor Visit Details & Journal

APPOINTMENT DATE: ___/___/___ (CONTINUED)

DOCTOR'S / PRACTITIONER'S INSTRUCTIONS, DIAGNOSIS & ACTION PLAN FOR ME

FOLLOW-UP APPOINTMENT DATE & TIME:

NEW MEDICATION(S):

FOLLOW-UP LAB TESTS:

FOLLOW-UP IMAGING:

MY REMINDERS / THOUGHTS / NOTES

My Doctor Visit Details & Journal

APPOINTMENT DATE: ___/___/___ *(CONTINUED)*

MY REMINDERS / THOUGHTS / NOTES

My Doctor Visit Details & Journal

NAME OF DOCTOR / PRACTITIONER: _____

MEDICAL SPECIALTY: _____ APPOINTMENT DATE & TIME: _____

REASON FOR VISIT: ○ FOLLOW UP ○ INITIAL CONSULT ○ OTHER _____

VITAL SIGNS: BP _____ PULSE / HR _____ TEMP _____ WEIGHT _____

TODAY'S SYMPTOMS / CONCERNS

LIST OF QUESTIONS TO ASK / TOPICS TO DISCUSS

QUESTION / TOPIC #1:

ANSWER TO #1:

QUESTION / TOPIC #2:

ANSWER TO #2:

My Doctor Visit Details & Journal

APPOINTMENT DATE: ___/___/___ (*CONTINUED*)

QUESTION / TOPIC #3:

ANSWER TO #3:

QUESTION / TOPIC #4:

ANSWER TO #4:

QUESTION / TOPIC #5:

ANSWER TO #5:

My Doctor Visit Details & Journal

APPOINTMENT DATE: ___/___/___ (CONTINUED)

DOCTOR'S / PRACTITIONER'S INSTRUCTIONS, DIAGNOSIS & ACTION PLAN FOR ME

FOLLOW-UP APPOINTMENT DATE & TIME:
_____
_____
_____

NEW MEDICATION(S):
_____
_____
_____

FOLLOW-UP LAB TESTS:
_____
_____

FOLLOW-UP IMAGING:
_____
_____
_____

MY REMINDERS / THOUGHTS / NOTES

_____
_____
_____
_____
_____
_____
_____
_____
_____
_____

My Doctor Visit Details & Journal

APPOINTMENT DATE: ___/___/___ (CONTINUED)

MY REMINDERS / THOUGHTS / NOTES

My Doctor Visit Details & Journal

NAME OF DOCTOR / PRACTITIONER: _____

MEDICAL SPECIALTY: _____ APPOINTMENT DATE & TIME: _____

REASON FOR VISIT: ○ FOLLOW UP   ○ INITIAL CONSULT   ○ OTHER _____

VITAL SIGNS: BP _____   PULSE / HR _____   TEMP _____   WEIGHT _____

TODAY'S SYMPTOMS / CONCERNS

_____

_____

LIST OF QUESTIONS TO ASK / TOPICS TO DISCUSS

QUESTION / TOPIC #1:

_____

_____

_____

ANSWER TO #1:

_____

_____

_____

QUESTION / TOPIC #2:

_____

_____

ANSWER TO #2:

_____

_____

_____

My Doctor Visit Details & Journal

APPOINTMENT DATE: ___/___/___ (*CONTINUED*)

QUESTION / TOPIC #3:

ANSWER TO #3:

QUESTION / TOPIC #4:

ANSWER TO #4:

QUESTION / TOPIC #5:

ANSWER TO #5:

My Doctor Visit Details & Journal

APPOINTMENT DATE: ___/___/___ (CONTINUED)

DOCTOR'S / PRACTITIONER'S INSTRUCTIONS, DIAGNOSIS & ACTION PLAN FOR ME

FOLLOW-UP APPOINTMENT DATE & TIME:

NEW MEDICATION(S):

FOLLOW-UP LAB TESTS:

FOLLOW-UP IMAGING:

MY REMINDERS / THOUGHTS / NOTES

My Doctor Visit Details & Journal

APPOINTMENT DATE: ___/___/___ (CONTINUED)

MY REMINDERS / THOUGHTS / NOTES

My Doctor Visit Details & Journal

NAME OF DOCTOR / PRACTITIONER: _____

MEDICAL SPECIALTY: _____ APPOINTMENT DATE & TIME: _____

REASON FOR VISIT: ○ FOLLOW UP ○ INITIAL CONSULT ○ OTHER _____

VITAL SIGNS: BP _____ PULSE / HR _____ TEMP _____ WEIGHT _____

TODAY'S SYMPTOMS / CONCERNS

_____

_____

LIST OF QUESTIONS TO ASK / TOPICS TO DISCUSS

QUESTION / TOPIC #1:

_____

_____

_____

ANSWER TO #1:

_____

_____

QUESTION / TOPIC #2:

_____

_____

ANSWER TO #2:

_____

_____

My Doctor Visit Details & Journal

APPOINTMENT DATE: ___/___/___ (CONTINUED)

QUESTION / TOPIC #3:

ANSWER TO #3:

QUESTION / TOPIC #4:

ANSWER TO #4:

QUESTION / TOPIC #5:

ANSWER TO #5:

My Doctor Visit Details & Journal

APPOINTMENT DATE: ___/___/___ (CONTINUED)

DOCTOR'S / PRACTITIONER'S INSTRUCTIONS, DIAGNOSIS & ACTION PLAN FOR ME

FOLLOW-UP APPOINTMENT DATE & TIME:

NEW MEDICATION(S):

FOLLOW-UP LAB TESTS:

FOLLOW-UP IMAGING:

MY REMINDERS / THOUGHTS / NOTES

My Doctor Visit Details & Journal

APPOINTMENT DATE: ___/___/___ (*CONTINUED*)

MY REMINDERS / THOUGHTS / NOTES

My Doctor Visit Details & Journal

NAME OF DOCTOR / PRACTITIONER: _____

MEDICAL SPECIALTY: _____ APPOINTMENT DATE & TIME: _____

REASON FOR VISIT: ○ FOLLOW UP ○ INITIAL CONSULT ○ OTHER _____

VITAL SIGNS: BP _____ PULSE / HR _____ TEMP _____ WEIGHT _____

TODAY'S SYMPTOMS / CONCERNS

_____

_____

LIST OF QUESTIONS TO ASK / TOPICS TO DISCUSS

QUESTION / TOPIC #1:

_____

_____

_____

ANSWER TO #1:

_____

_____

QUESTION / TOPIC #2:

_____

_____

ANSWER TO #2:

_____

_____

My Doctor Visit Details & Journal

APPOINTMENT DATE: ___/___/___ (*CONTINUED*)

QUESTION / TOPIC #3:

ANSWER TO #3:

QUESTION / TOPIC #4:

ANSWER TO #4: ,

QUESTION / TOPIC #5:

ANSWER TO #5:

My Doctor Visit Details & Journal

APPOINTMENT DATE: ___/___/___ (*CONTINUED*)

DOCTOR'S / PRACTITIONER'S INSTRUCTIONS, DIAGNOSIS & ACTION PLAN FOR ME

FOLLOW-UP APPOINTMENT DATE & TIME:

NEW MEDICATION(S):

FOLLOW-UP LAB TESTS:

FOLLOW-UP IMAGING:

MY REMINDERS / THOUGHTS / NOTES

My Doctor Visit Details & Journal

APPOINTMENT DATE: ___/___/___ (*CONTINUED*)

MY REMINDERS / THOUGHTS / NOTES

My Doctor Visit Details & Journal

NAME OF DOCTOR / PRACTITIONER: _____

MEDICAL SPECIALTY: _____ APPOINTMENT DATE & TIME: _____

REASON FOR VISIT: ○ FOLLOW UP   ○ INITIAL CONSULT   ○ OTHER _____

VITAL SIGNS: BP _____ PULSE / HR _____ TEMP _____ WEIGHT _____

TODAY'S SYMPTOMS / CONCERNS

_____

_____

LIST OF QUESTIONS TO ASK / TOPICS TO DISCUSS

QUESTION / TOPIC #1:

_____

_____

_____

ANSWER TO #1:

_____

_____

_____

QUESTION / TOPIC #2:

_____

_____

ANSWER TO #2:

_____

_____

_____

My Doctor Visit Details & Journal

APPOINTMENT DATE: ___/___/___ (CONTINUED)

QUESTION / TOPIC #3:

_____

_____

_____

ANSWER TO #3:

_____

_____

_____

QUESTION / TOPIC #4:

_____

_____

_____

ANSWER TO #4:

_____

_____

_____

QUESTION / TOPIC #5:

_____

_____

_____

ANSWER TO #5:

_____

_____

_____

My Doctor Visit Details & Journal

APPOINTMENT DATE: ___/___/___ (CONTINUED)

DOCTOR'S / PRACTITIONER'S INSTRUCTIONS, DIAGNOSIS & ACTION PLAN FOR ME

FOLLOW-UP APPOINTMENT DATE & TIME:
_____
_____
_____

NEW MEDICATION(S):
_____
_____
_____

FOLLOW-UP LAB TESTS:
_____
_____
_____

FOLLOW-UP IMAGING:
_____
_____
_____

MY REMINDERS / THOUGHTS / NOTES

_____
_____
_____
_____
_____
_____
_____
_____
_____
_____

My Doctor Visit Details & Journal

APPOINTMENT DATE: ___/___/___ (CONTINUED)

MY REMINDERS / THOUGHTS / NOTES

My Doctor Visit Details & Journal

NAME OF DOCTOR / PRACTITIONER: _____

MEDICAL SPECIALTY: _____ APPOINTMENT DATE & TIME: _____

REASON FOR VISIT: ○ FOLLOW UP   ○ INITIAL CONSULT   ○ OTHER _____

VITAL SIGNS: BP _____ PULSE / HR _____ TEMP _____ WEIGHT _____

TODAY'S SYMPTOMS / CONCERNS

_____

_____

LIST OF QUESTIONS TO ASK / TOPICS TO DISCUSS

QUESTION / TOPIC #1:

_____

_____

_____

ANSWER TO #1:

_____

_____

_____

QUESTION / TOPIC #2:

_____

_____

ANSWER TO #2:

_____

_____

_____

My Doctor Visit Details & Journal

APPOINTMENT DATE: ___/___/___ (CONTINUED)

QUESTION / TOPIC #3:

ANSWER TO #3:

QUESTION / TOPIC #4:

ANSWER TO #4:

QUESTION / TOPIC #5:

ANSWER TO #5:

My Doctor Visit Details & Journal

APPOINTMENT DATE: ___/___/___ (CONTINUED)

DOCTOR'S / PRACTITIONER'S INSTRUCTIONS, DIAGNOSIS & ACTION PLAN FOR ME

FOLLOW-UP APPOINTMENT DATE & TIME:

NEW MEDICATION(S):

FOLLOW-UP LAB TESTS:

FOLLOW-UP IMAGING:

MY REMINDERS / THOUGHTS / NOTES

My Doctor Visit Details & Journal

APPOINTMENT DATE: ___/___/___ (CONTINUED)

MY REMINDERS / THOUGHTS / NOTES

My Doctor Visit Details & Journal

NAME OF DOCTOR / PRACTITIONER: _____

MEDICAL SPECIALTY: _____ APPOINTMENT DATE & TIME: _____

REASON FOR VISIT: ○ FOLLOW UP ○ INITIAL CONSULT ○ OTHER _____

VITAL SIGNS: BP _____ PULSE / HR _____ TEMP _____ WEIGHT _____

TODAY'S SYMPTOMS / CONCERNS

_____

_____

LIST OF QUESTIONS TO ASK / TOPICS TO DISCUSS

QUESTION / TOPIC #1:

_____

_____

_____

ANSWER TO #1:

_____

_____

_____

QUESTION / TOPIC #2:

_____

_____

ANSWER TO #2:

_____

_____

_____

My Doctor Visit Details & Journal

APPOINTMENT DATE: ___/___/___ *(CONTINUED)*

QUESTION / TOPIC #3:

_____

_____

_____

ANSWER TO #3:

_____

_____

_____

QUESTION / TOPIC #4:

_____

_____

_____

ANSWER TO #4:

_____

_____

_____

QUESTION / TOPIC #5:

_____

_____

_____

ANSWER TO #5:

_____

_____

_____

My Doctor Visit Details & Journal

APPOINTMENT DATE: ___/___/___ (CONTINUED)

DOCTOR'S / PRACTITIONER'S INSTRUCTIONS, DIAGNOSIS & ACTION PLAN FOR ME

FOLLOW-UP APPOINTMENT DATE & TIME:

NEW MEDICATION(S):

FOLLOW-UP LAB TESTS:

FOLLOW-UP IMAGING:

MY REMINDERS / THOUGHTS / NOTES

My Doctor Visit Details & Journal

APPOINTMENT DATE: ___/___/___ (*CONTINUED*)

MY REMINDERS / THOUGHTS / NOTES

A Special Message from Olivia Davenport, Author
My Doctor Appointment Log Book & Journal

As a thank you for your purchase of this book, I am giving my readers a free *Medical Records Release* form to request your medical records from current and previous physicians and hospitals.

As I state in the book, it's always a good idea to have a copy of your most recent medical records on hand, especially if you're planning to move or change doctors.

This form is an Adobe portable document format (pdf) file, which can be printed and filled out in writing or edited and saved on your computer (for personal use only, please).

Download it from the Cabin Creek Publishing website, here:

https://cabincreekpublishing.com/download-from-olivia-davenport/

I hope the book and this gifted *Medical Records Release* form download are helpful to you!

All the best,

Olivia

Olivia

About the Author

Author Olivia Davenport wants to help patients work better with their doctors and other medical practitioners. As a Lupus patient and a breast cancer survivor, she is treated by all types of doctors—from her family physician and rheumatologist to her surgeons, radiologists, and oncologists, just to name a few.

With ongoing multiple appointments with many different practitioners, she quickly realized that the only way to manage her care successfully was to get organized and develop a way to keep track of it all. This book, *My Doctor Appointment Log Book and Journal: The Patient's Tool to Prepare for and Record What Happens at Every Doctor Visit*, is the result of her own research and self-discovery about how best to manage her doctor visits and overall medical care. Olivia is eager to share this book and what she has learned, knowing that many patients could benefit from it.

Olivia is the author of two other books:
- *Live a Beautiful Life with Lupus: Habits and Rituals for Thriving with an Autoimmune Disease—Body, Mind, and Spirit* (available in print and Kindle e-book formats)
- *Lupus Diary: Tracking Your Life with Lupus—Body, Mind, and Spirit* is the companion to her first book (available in print format only)

Olivia lives in northern Nevada with her husband and their odd-eyed cat, Kitty-Witty.

www.ingramcontent.com/pod-product-compliance
Lightning Source LLC
Chambersburg PA
CBHW080557030426
42336CB00019B/3230